BAKING

DEMYSTIFIED

50 Easy And Delicious Grain-Free And Gluten-Free Baking Recipes

(Weight watchers Book 2)

BY

VIRGINIA A. CALDWELL

E-book Edition

First published in 2016

ISBN-13: 978-1537250151

ISBN-10: 1537250159

Contents

For more of my awesome cookbooks and recipes please visit my author central page:

amazon.com/author/virginiacaldwell

Salty Baked Whole Sea Trout

Ingredients

- 3 pounds coarse natural sea salt
- 2 sea trout, scaled and cleaned
- Large bunch fresh fennel fronds and stalks
- Freshly ground black pepper and Sea salt

Preparation

1. Preheat the oven to about 400 degrees F.

2. Rub pepper and salt into the insides of the sea trout, and cram the unsliced fennel fronds and stalks into the gut cavity.

3. Spread a layer of salt about 1/2-inch deep on the bottom of a large roasting tin. Lay the trout on the salt. Spread the remaining salt on the fish till it is fully covered to about 1/2-inch thick. Don't bother if the head and tail sticks out a little. Shower some water over the salt.

4. Bake for about 40 to 45 minutes. To check if the fish is done, prick with a spit and if it comes out warm the fish is ready. Remove the salt crust, as well as the skin too.

Creamy Sweet Potato Orange Pie

Ingredients

• 1 (10-inch) tart shell or Pastry Pie Dough for 1 (9-inch) pie pan

• 6 large eggs

• 3 cups boiled sweet potatoes, skinned, cooked, drained and mashed

• 2 oranges, juiced

• 1½ cup light brown sugar

• 1 stick unsalted butter, dissolved

• 1¼ cup heavy cream

• 1 teaspoon allspice

• 1 teaspoon cinnamon

• ½ teaspoon fresh grated nutmeg

PASTRY DOUGH RECIPE:

14 ounces cold chopped butter

5 cups flour

1 cup ice water

3 teaspoons salt

Preparation

1. Bake the tart shells for about 10 minutes in a preheated 350 degree oven. Mix together the ingredients in a mixing

bowl, completely. Pour the sweet potato mixture into the tart shell and place in the 350 degree oven and bake for another 25 minutes or until the middle becomes set.

2. Mix together the butter, flour, salt and pulse in a mixing bowl until the mixture becomes very coarse. Transfer the flour and butter mixture into a big mixing bowl and pour in the ice water. Pour into a clean, flat surface. Using the palm of your hand, gradually push and pull the mixture to mould it into dough. Do not knead the dough only slightly pressing it.

Baked Salmon with Truffles in Puff Pastry

Ingredients

• 3 pounds salmon fillet sliced from the middle of the a side of salmon, boned and skinned

• 4 hard cooked eggs, diced

• 3 tablespoons flat-leaf parsley, shredded

• 1 pound puff pastry, thawed

• 3 bunches watercress, for garnish

• 1 ounce black truffles, chopped

• 2 eggs, whisked

• Salt and pepper

Preparation

1. Preheat the oven to about 400 degrees F.

2. Slice the puff pastry into 2 uniform sizes a bit bigger than your salmon. Lay 1 piece of pastry on the cookie sheet which lined with parchment paper or oiled and set the side of salmon on it. Garnish with parsley. Arrange the chopped black truffles on the salmon like scales and cover as much as possible. Top the truffles with the diced hard boiled eggs and spice with salt and pepper.

3. Lay the second piece of pastry on the first and seal the edges and tuck with your fingers. Use egg wash to brush the top and bake for about half an hour until the pastry turns

golden brown. Allow it to cool for about 10 minutes and then divide into 6 uniform sizes, garnish the plate with the watercress and serve.

Cornbread And Sweet Potato

Ingredients

- 10 tablespoons butter, dissolved
- 1½ cup all-purpose flour
- 3 cups cornmeal
- 1 teaspoon baking soda
- 1¼ tablespoon baking powder
- 2 cups buttermilk
- 1 teaspoon pumpkin pie spice
- 5 eggs, room temperature
- 1¼ cup mashed sweet potatoes
- ½ cup honey
- ½ cup brown sugar
- 1¼ teaspoon salt

Preparations

1. Preheat the oven to about 35o degrees F.

2. Combine the flour, cornmeal, brown sugar, baking soda, salt, baking powder and pumpkin pie spice in a big mixing bowl.

3. Using another medium mixing bowl, combine the eggs, mashed sweet potatoes, buttermilk, butter and honey. Stir the wet ingredients into the bowl of dry ingredients, and whisk until completely blended.

4. Decant the batter into a cast-iron skillet and use a spatula to make it smooth to a uniform layer. Put in the oven and bake for about half an hour or until it turns a golden brown color and a toothpick dipped into the middle comes out clean. Serve the cornbread.

Chocolate Coconut Chips

Ingredients

- 4 cups flaked coconut
- 3 sticks unsalted butter, melted
- 3 cups chocolate chips
- ¾ cup packed light brown sugar
- 3 large eggs
- ¾ cup white sugar
- 2 teaspoons pure vanilla extract
- 3 tablespoons milk
- 2½ cups all-purpose flour
- 1¼ teaspoon baking soda melted in 3 teaspoons hot water
- ¾ teaspoon ground cinnamon
- ¾ tablespoon salt
- 1½ cup dried cherries (snip into halves with kitchen scissors)

Preparation

1. Preheat the oven to about 350 degrees F.

2. Mix together the butter and sugars and whisk until fluffy and light. Whisk in the eggs, one by one. Pour in the vanilla, milk and baking soda mixture. Mix together the salt, flour and cinnamon and gently stir it into the butter mixture. Add the chocolate chips, coconut and cherries.

3. Line the baking sheets with parchment paper and drop mounds of dough onto it. Bake for about 15 minutes or until the edges are fairly browned. Allow it to cool for 5 minutes.

Fried Chicken With Coleslaw

Ingredients

- 10 chicken parts, like thighs, breasts and drumsticks
- Oil, for shallow frying
- 4 ounces all-purpose flour
- 2½ cups buttermilk
- 3 tablespoons sweet paprika
- 2¼ teaspoons chile powder
- 4½ teaspoons table salt
- 3 tablespoons smoked paprika
- 2½ teaspoons dried basil
- 2 ounces cornstarch
- 2½ teaspoons dried marjoram
- 3 teaspoons garlic powder
- 3 teaspoons ground dried oregano
- 2½ teaspoons ground white pepper
- 2¼ teaspoons ground dried sage
- Coleslaw, for serving
- 3 teaspoons onion salt

Preparation

1. Arrange the chicken in a big mixing bowl, top with the buttermilk and freeze for about 12 hours.

2. Preheat the oven to around 375 degrees F. Combine the smoked paprika, flour, sweet paprika, basil, salt, cornstarch, chili powder, sage, garlic powder, onion salt, marjoram, oregano, and white pepper in a baking dish or big bowl.

3. Heat the oil in a big frying pan over medium-low heat. Take the chicken one piece at a time out of the buttermilk, shake off any surplus and toss it in the flour mixture. Deep-fry the chicken for about 6 to 7 minutes a side, about 2 or 3 pieces at a time, until it turns a golden brown and is done. Drain off excess oil on paper towels, then place on a baking sheet and bake for another 15 minutes.

4. Serve the chicken with some coleslaw.

Sun-Dried Tomato And Corn Muffin

Ingredients

- 4 medium eggs

- 2 (9-ounce) packs corn muffin mix

- 1 cup chopped sun-dried tomatoes

- 2½ cups frozen whole kernel corn, defrosted

- ¾ cup buttermilk

- 4 garlic cloves, chopped

- ¾ cup sour cream

Preparation

1. Preheat the oven to about 375 degrees F. Rub grease into 2 muffin tins.

2. Mix together the corn, muffin mix, sun-dried tomatoes and garlic in a bowl. Whisk to mix properly. Using a small mixing bowl combine the sour cream, buttermilk, and eggs until properly mixed. Stir the buttermilk mixture into the bowl of muffin mix. Whisk to mix properly. Pour the mix into the muffin tins, pouring them half full. Bake for about 15 to 20 minutes or until it takes a golden brown color on top.

Baked Sugary Apples

Ingredients

- 5 tablespoons light brown sugar

- 3 Golden Delicious apples

- Powdered cinnamon, for sprinkling

- Creamy Custard Sauce

- 3 tablespoons butter

- **Creamy custard sauce:**

- 3 egg yolks

- 1 pint light vanilla ice cream, melted

Preparation

1. Preheat the oven to 350 degrees.

2. Rinse and dry the apples. Chop the apples into two and get rid of the core but leave the stems whole. Arrange the apples in a baking dish. Split the butter into each core space. Sprinkle a dash of cinnamon and a tablespoon of sugar on each apple half.

3. Bake the apples for half an hour until the skin becomes soft and bubbly. Serve with Creamy Custard Sauce.

4. Next, heat the dissolved ice cream in a little saucepan over low heat until it is hot. Whisk the yolks in a small mixing bowl until smooth. While whisking the egg, gently pour 2 tablespoons of hot dissolved ice cream into the yolks and mix together. While whisking repeatedly, gently add the

remaining hot liquid to the yolk mixture. Transfer the mixture into the pan and place on low heat.

Baked Kale with Vinegar Chips

Ingredients

- 1¼ bunch kale, stemmed, washed, dried
- ½ cup olive oil
- Enough quantity cider vinegar
- Sea salt

Preparation

1. Preparing the kale chips: Preheat the oven to about 350 degrees F. Pour in the kale and oil and kale into a plastic bag. Close the bag and swirl the oil around as uniformly as possible to soak the kale. Arrange the kale on a baking tray and sauté for about 10 to 15 minutes until it turns crispy.

2. Sprinkle with sea salt and cider vinegar. Serve and enjoy.

Baked Apple And Oat Muffins

Ingredients

- 2 big eggs, lightly whisked
- 3 cups old-fashioned or quick-cooking oats
- 3 tablespoons vegetable oil
- 1 cup packed brown sugar
- 1½ cups all-purpose flour
- 3 teaspoons baking powder
- 1 teaspoon salt
- 1 teaspoon baking soda
- 1¼ cup buttermilk
- ¾ teaspoons ground cinnamon
- ¾ cup walnuts, diced
- 1 cup Golden Delicious or Granny Smith apples, shredded

Preparation

1. Preheat the oven to about 400 degrees F.

2. Rub oil into a 12-inch standard muffin pan cups. Mix together the oats, sugar, flour, baking powder, salt, baking soda, and ground cinnamon in a medium mixing bowl.

3. Using another mixing bowl, whisk the buttermilk, egg and oil, until well combined; add in the diced apples. Pour the apple mixture into the bowl of flour mixture, and whisk

until the flour mixture is moistened and the batter very thick. Whisk in the diced walnuts.

4. Scoop the batter into ready muffin-pan cups. Bake for about 20 to 25 minutes or until the muffins start to brown and a toothpick dipped in the middle of muffins comes out clean. Take the muffins out of the pan. Serve warm, or allow it to cool on wire rack and serve later.

Chewy Buttermilk Cookies

Ingredients

- 2 large eggs
- 3 cups all-purpose flour
- ¾ teaspoon baking powder
- 2 teaspoons baking soda
- 2 cups white sugar
- 1¼ cup dissolved butter
- 4 tablespoons buttermilk
- 1¼ teaspoon vanilla extract
- Sprinkles or colored sugar, for garnishing

Preparation

1. Preheat oven to 375 degrees F.

2. Combine the baking soda, flour, and baking powder in a small mixing bowl. Leave to stand.

3. Whisk together the butter and sugar in a medium mixing bowl until it becomes smooth. Whisk in the vanilla and egg. Gently stir in the dry ingredients and pour in sufficient buttermilk to dampen the dough and make it tender, not wet.

4. Mold rounded teaspoons of dough into balls and arrange them on an ungreased cookie sheet. Using your brush or fingers, dampen the top of each cookie with the rest of the

buttermilk and gently flatten the top of each cookie. Garnish with colored sprinkles or raw sugar.

5. Allow to bake for about 8 to 10 minutes or until it is fairly golden and leave it to stand for another 2 minutes before transferring to a rack to cool.

Glazed Bourbon Chicken Wings

Ingredients

• 1 (12 ounces) can frozen apple juice concentrate, defrosted

• 2 lbs chicken wings, spruced

• ¾ cup soy sauce

• 1½ cup Maker's Mark (R) Bourbon

• ½ cup cider vinegar

• 6 medium cloves garlic, chopped

• ½ cup dark brown sugar

• ½ teaspoons grated red pepper

• Chopped scallions and apples, for garnish

• 1¼ tablespoon maple syrup

• 1½ teaspoon salt

Preparation

1. Mix together all the ingredients in a medium-sized pot. Allow it to boil on high heat and then lower heat to a simmer for about half an hour or until the wings become tender and the glaze has thickened, coating the wings.

2. Preheat the oven to about 325 degrees F. Take the wings out of the pot and place on a sheet tray lined with parchment. Bake for roughly 15 to 20 minutes or until the

wings start to color and the glaze turns shiny. Top with chopped scallions and apple. Serve at once.

Baked Cheesy Tortellini Sauce

Ingredients

- 1 recipe Bolognese Sauce

- 1 pound cheese tortellini, boiled

- 1½ teaspoon butter

- 1¼ cup Parmigiano-Reggiano cheese, shredded

Preparation

Preheat the oven to about 425 degrees F. Rub butter on a ceramic gratin dish. Flip the pasta with the salt, olive oil, and pepper. Arrange the pasta at the bottom of the dish. Scoop the sauce and sprinkle over the pasta. Top the sauce with the shredded cheese. Put in the oven and bake for approximately 8 to 12 minutes or until the cheese becomes golden brown and bouncy.

Baked Cheesy Grits

Ingredients

- 3 eggs, whisked
- 4 cups boiled grits
- Paprika, to taste
- 2 cups evaporated milk
- 3 tablespoons dissolved butter
- 2 dashes Cayenne pepper, to taste
- 2 cups Cheddar, shredded

Preparation

1. Preheat the oven to about 400 degrees.

2. Squash the grits until completely smooth. Pour in dissolved butter, evaporated milk and eggs. Add 2 cups of shredded cheese, reserving half a cup for the topping. Mix completely. Stir in the cayenne and paprika. Pour the mixture into a buttered casserole. Bake for about half an hour or until it turns brown. Garnish with the rest of the shredded cheese and extra paprika. Place in the oven and heat for a couple more minutes or until the topping has dissolved.

Bakers Blueberry Cornbread

Ingredients

- 3 cups milk
- 12 tablespoons dissolved unsalted butter
- 5 eggs
- 3½ cups all-purpose flour
- 1¼ cup blue cornmeal
- 2 cups sugar
- 2½ tablespoons baking powder
- 3 pints blueberries
- 1 cup vegetable oil
- 1½ teaspoon salt

Preparation

1. Preheat the oven to about 325 degrees F. Grease a 12-inch skillet generously with butter. Combine the baking powder, flour, blue cornmeal, sugar, and salt together in a mixing bowl. Combine the vegetable oil, milk, and 6 tablespoons dissolved butter. Stir the wet ingredients into the bowl of dry ingredients. Add 1 pint of blueberries. Pour the batter into the skillet and garnish with the rest of the blueberries.

Bake for about 1 hour or until the top cracks and a toothpick inserted comes out clean. Take tray out of the oven, pierce several holes with the skewer and brush the rest of the dissolved butter and allow it to cool.

Buttery Pumpkin Bread

Ingredients

- 1 pound unsalted butter, dissolved
- 12 eggs
- 2 pounds canned pumpkin
- 6 cups flour
- 6 cups buttermilk
- 4 cups sugar
- 6 cups cornmeal (yellow or white)
- 3 tablespoons baking soda
- 2 ½ tablespoons baking powder
- 2 tablespoons salt
- Dash ground nutmeg
- ¾ teaspoon cinnamon

Preparation

1. Preheat the oven to about 350 degrees F. Rub grease into 7 regular muffin tins.

2. Combine the eggs, sugar, pumpkin and buttermilk until well mixed and leave to stand. Using another bowl, blend together all the dry ingredients. Stir the pumpkin mixture into the bowl of dry ingredients, mixing properly. Whisk in the dissolved butter.

3. Transfer 3 ounces of batter in each muffin cup and place on the pan. Bake for about 15 to 20 minutes or until a toothpick inserted in the middle comes out clean.

Sweet Bacon Soufflé

Ingredients

- 4 big eggs
- 4 pounds sweet potatoes, baked and still warm
- 4 tablespoons light brown sugar

4 tablespoons unsalted butter, dissolved

- Kosher salt and freshly ground black pepper
- 3 ounces cream cheese, room temperature

TOPPING:

6 slices bacon, boiled and shredded

1 cup light brown sugar

½ cup all-purpose flour

¾ cup pecans, diced

4 tablespoons unsalted butter, refrigerated, diced

Preparation

1. Preheat the oven to about 350 degrees F.

2. Skin the sweet potatoes and place the skin in a bowl. Whisk in the butter using a stand mixer or a hand mixer until well blended. Stir in the brown sugar, cream cheese and eggs, one at a time. Season with pepper and salt.

3. To prepare the topping: combine the pecans, brown sugar, butter, flour and bacon in another bowl until it is crumbly.

4. Pour the mixture into a deep-dish pie plate and bake for half an hour until it is puffed and golden brown. Leave to stand for about 10 minutes before serving.

Lime-Spiced Baked Chicken Wings

Ingredients

- 8 pounds chicken wings
- 3 large garlic cloves, diced
- 2 habaneros, seeded and diced
- 3 teaspoons allspice
- ½ cup soy sauce
- ½ cup brown sugar
- ½ cup honey
- 1½ teaspoon ground ginger
- 3 teaspoons fennel seed
- 3 tablespoons sugar

3 teaspoons dried thyme

- 3 teaspoons cayenne pepper
- 3 large green onions, sliced
- ½ cup lime juice
- ½ cup apple cider vinegar
- ½ cup orange juice

Preparation

1. Blend all the ingredients aside from the chicken together in a food processor until its smooth. Preserve 1 cup of marinade. Put the chicken wings into a big sealable plastic

bag and pour in the rest of the marinade on them. Seal and marinate in the refrigerator for about 4 to 6 hours.

2. Preheat the oven to about 350 degrees F. use parchment paper to line the inside of 2 sheet trays. Take out the chicken from the bag and put it on the baking sheets. Bake for approximately 20 minutes. Next, boil the preserved marinade in a small saucepan. Boil for about 12 minutes or until it thickens a bit. After about 20 to 25 minutes, take the chicken out of the oven. Brush the chicken with the glaze. Increase the heat to about 400 degrees F and boil the chicken until it's done.

Baked Leftover Pizza Pies

Ingredients

- Mozzarella
- Leftover Chinese food
- Leftover pizza
- Water

Preparation

1. Preheat the oven to about 425 degrees F.

Scatter the leftover Chinese food uniformly on top of the pizza. Drizzle a thin layer of cheese on it. Begin at the crust end and roll the pizza into a thick pinwheel. Use toothpicks to pin down the rolls and place on the baking sheet. Bake for about 10 minutes or until it becomes crispy. Serve.

Oven Baked Crusty Pumpkin Cheesecake

Ingredients

CRUST:

- 3½ tablespoons light brown sugar
- 2 cups graham cracker crumbs
- 1 stick dissolved salted butter
- ¾ teaspoon ground cinnamon

FILLING:

1 (15-ounce) can puréed pumpkin

3 tablespoons all-purpose flour

4 (8-ounce) packs cream cheese, at room temperature

½ cup sour cream

4 large eggs with 1 egg yolk

¾ teaspoon ground cinnamon

2 cups sugar

¼ teaspoon ground cloves

¼ teaspoon fresh ground nutmeg

1½ teaspoon vanilla extract

Preparation

Preheat the oven to about 350 degrees F.

For crust:

1. Mix together the crumbs, cinnamon and sugar in a medium-sized mixing bowl. Stir in the dissolved butter. Press down flat into a 9-inch spring form pan. Leave to stand.

For filling:

1. Whisk the cream cheese until it becomes smooth. Stir in the pumpkin puree, egg yolk, sour cream, eggs, sugar and other spices. Pour in the vanilla and flour. Stir them together until well blended.

2. Pour the mixture into the crust. Spread out uniformly and put in the oven for about an hour. Take the tray out of the oven and leave to cool for about 15 minutes. Wrap in plastic wrap and freeze for about 4 hours.

Baked Fillet Cardoons

Ingredients

• 5 anchovy fillets, washed, dried, and finely chopped

• 25 stalks cardoons, rinsed, cooked and dried

• 5 tablespoons extra-virgin olive oil, with extra for greasing the pan

• ½ cup shredded caciocavallo, with ½ cup medium chopped

• 1 cup fresh bread crumbs

• ½ cup freshly ground pecorino, with 1 cup cubed

• 1 bunch freshly diced Italian parsley leaves

• 1 lemon, juiced, for garnish

• Salt and freshly grated black pepper

Preparation

1. Preheat the oven to about 350 degrees F.

2. Lightly rub grease into a shallow 9 by 13-inch grating dish. Place the cardoons in a single layer on the bottom of the pan. Top the cardoons with ½ cup shredded caciocavallo, ½ cup shredded pecorino, crumbs and parsley and add the anchovies, chopped pecorino and chopped caciocavallo on top.

3. Season with the pepper and salt to taste. Stir in 4 tablespoons of olive oil and mix well.

4. Sprinkle the rest 1 tablespoon of olive oil on top. Put tray in the oven and bake for about 30 minutes or until the top turn golden brown. Serve while hot with squeeze of lemon.

Baked Barbeque Bean Sauce

Ingredients

- ¾ cup BBQ sauce

- 4 (1-pound) cans baked beans

- 2 large green onions, thinly sliced

- 8 strips of bacon, boiled and diced

- ¾ cup brown sugar

Preparation

1. Preheat the oven to about 350 degrees F.

2. Combine the BBQ sauce, beans, and bacon, sugar and green onions together in a baking dish, cover using foil and bake for roughly half an hour. Serve!

Oven-Baked Honey Yams

Ingredients

- 5 big yams
- 1 cup honey
- 3 tablespoons unsalted butter, cut into pieces
- 1¼ tablespoon ground allspice
- 3 tablespoons powdered cinnamon
- 1½ tablespoon ground nutmeg
- 1½ tablespoon brown sugar

Preparation

1. Preheat the oven to about 350 degrees F. Cook the yams for about 20 to 30 minutes in sufficient water until it is almost soft. Drain the yams out of the water and cool for a while. Peel and slice into big sizes.

2. Place the yams in a baking dish. Garnish with the butter and drizzle with the cinnamon, brown sugar, allspice, and nutmeg. Sprinkle the honey on top. Bake for about 15 to 20 minutes or until the yams are done and the top starts to turn brown.

Creamy Baked Pot Eggs

Ingredients

• 5 free-range eggs

• 7 ounces crème fraiche

• Dash nutmeg

• Red lumpfish roe, for garnish, optional

• Handful of diced dill, with some little sprigs, for garnish, optional

• Freshly ground black pepper and salt

Preparation

1. Preheat the oven to around 350 degrees F.

2. Spice the crème fraiche with freshly ground pepper, salt and a dash of nutmeg.

3. Pour a heaped tablespoon of crème fraiche into the bottom of a ramekin, add a little diced dill. Break an egg into the mixture, stir in a second tablespoon of crème fraiche and season with a dash each of salt, nutmeg and pepper. Do the same with 3 more ramekins.

4. Put the ramekins in a baking dish and sprinkle sufficient warm water into the dish to fill it halfway up the sides of the ramekins. Bake for about 15 minutes, or until the egg yolks become set as you prefer.

5. If you desire, you can top off each serving with a teaspoon of red lumpfish roe and a sprig or two of dill.

Roasted Potato And Paprika Fries

Ingredients

- 5 big russet potatoes, washed, but not skinned
- Freshly grated black pepper
- 4 tablespoons olive oil
- Pinch steak spice seasoning
- Dash smoked paprika
- Dash sea salt

Preparation

1. Heat the oven to about 425 degrees F.

2. Slice the potatoes into equal thick 'hand cut fry slices' and place them in a big bowl filled with cold water. This can be done beforehand about 24 hours before use. It assists in removing surplus starch.

3. Drain the potatoes from the water and dry them with paper towels. Place them in a single layer on a baking sheet. Sprinkle oil, salt, paprika and pepper over them. Bake for half an hour or until they become tender with golden crispy edges.

4. Remove from the oven; garnish them with some dashes of steak spice.

Baked Buttery Mamaliga

Ingredients

- 1¼ tablespoon unsalted butter
- 2 cups water
- 1 pound kashkaval cheese, shredded
- 2 cups milk
- 2 tablespoons extra virgin olive oil
- 3 ears corn, kernels removed
- 1¼ cup cornmeal polenta, medium grind
- Salt and pepper

Preparation

Allow the water and milk to boil. Pour in the cornmeal and reduce heat to a simmer. Repeatedly stir for about 4 minutes until it becomes smooth. Whisk in half the cheese, 1½ tablespoon of the olive oil, the butter, the fresh corn and seasoning until the cheese has dissolved. Rub grease into a casserole with the rest of the olive oil and stir in the corn mixture. Garnish with the rest of the cheese and bake in an oven preheated to 400 degree until all the cheese dissolves and turns brown on top. Serve.

Cheesy Baked Shrimp with Tomatoes

Ingredients

- 2 pounds large shrimp, skinned and deveined

- 2 tablespoons olive oil

- 3 (14.5-ounce) cans of salt-less chopped tomatoes, with their juices

- 1 large onion, chopped

- ½ cup thinly chopped fresh flat-leaf parsley

- 3 cloves garlic, chopped

- 2 tablespoons thinly chopped fresh dill

- 1 cup feta cheese, shredded

- ½ teaspoon freshly grated black pepper

- ½ teaspoon salt

Preparation

1. Preheat the oven to about 400 degrees F.

2. Pour the oil into an oven proof skillet and heat over a medium-high heat. Stir in the onion and sauté for about 2 to 5 minutes, stirring, until tender, then pour in the garlic and stir for another 1 minute. Pour in the tomatoes and allow it to boil. Lower the heat to medium-low heat and allow it to simmer for approximately 5 minutes, until the tomato juices become thick.

3. Turn off the heat. Whisk in the dill, parsley, and shrimp and add a little salt and pepper for taste. Top with the feta cheese. Bake for about 12 minutes until the shrimp are done and the cheese softens.

Lemon-spiced Madeleine

Ingredients

- 5 large eggs
- 1½ cup flour
- 2 tablespoons brown sugar
- ¾ teaspoon baking powder
- 1 cup butter
- 1½ tablespoon honey
- ¾ cup sugar
- Zest of 1 lemon
- Dash salt

Preparation

1. Grease Madeleine tins and arrange them in the freezer. Heat the oven to about 400 degrees F.

2. Sift the flour and baking powder together.

3. Dissolve the butter into a medium-sized pan and stir in the honey, sugar, and lemon zest. Slightly whisk the eggs, and pour them into the butter mixture. Beat and pour into the flour to make the batter smooth. Pour it into the molds and bake for about 12 minutes or until the cakes are golden around the edges, puffed up and done, and keep the door closed while cooking.

Fat-free Chocolate Cookies

Ingredients

- 3 cups quick-cooking or old-fashioned oats, raw
- ¾ cups packed brown sugar
- 1½ cups all-purpose flour
- ¾ cup granulated sugar
- 2 medium eggs
- 1 cup trans-fat free vegetable oil spread
- 2 medium egg whites
- 2 teaspoons baking soda
- 3 teaspoons vanilla extract
- 1¼ cup bittersweet or semisweet chocolate chips
- ¾ teaspoon salt

Preparation

1. Preheat the oven to about 375 degrees F.

2. Turn the mixer to medium-low speed and whisk the sugars and vegetable spread in a big mixing bowl until well combined, repeatedly using a rubber spatula to scrape the bowl. Stir in the eggs, vanilla and egg whites, and whisk until it becomes smooth. Stir in the baking soda, flour, and salt until blended.

3. Using a wooden spoon, whisk in the chocolate chips and oats until well mixed. Mould the dough into rounded

tablespoonfuls 2 inches apart on the ungreased cookie sheets. Bake for about 15 minutes or until it becomes golden. Bake in batches if necessary. Use a wide, metal spatula to remove the cookies to a wire rack where it is to cool.

Broccoli With Chicken Casserole

Ingredients

• 1 pack chicken flavored Ramen noodles, shredded

• 1 cup mayonnaise

• 14 ounces chopped mushrooms, deep-fry in 2 tablespoon butter

• 1¾ cup sharp cheddar cheese, shredded

• 1 cup plain yogurt

• 3 large eggs

• Flavor Pack from Ramen

• ½ cup blue cheese dressing

• 7 cups broccoli, removed stems and heads, sliced and rinsed in salted water

• 2 teaspoon fresh grated black pepper

• 1 teaspoon salt

Preparation

1. Preheat the oven to about 375 degrees F.

2. Mix together the yogurt, mayonnaise, cheddar cheese; eggs, blue cheese dressing, pepper, salt, and flavor pack from noodles in a large mixing bowl. Using another bowl mix together the broccoli, broken noodles and mushrooms, then stir together the wet mixture with the vegetables to coat uniformly. Transfer to a nonstick spray coated 8 by 8-

inch baking dish, place cover and boil for 45 minutes. Then uncover and bake for another 15 minutes till it turns brown. Allow to cool for about 15 minutes before serving.

Baked Scottish Bread

Ingredients

- 6 cups sifted all-purpose flour
- 1 pound butter, melted
- ¾ teaspoon salt
- 1¼ cup sugar

Preparation

1. Preheat the oven to about 375 degrees F.

2. Start by whisking the butter and sugar together in a big mixing bowl. Stir in the salt to the first cup of flour and combine with the butter mixture by whisking with a wooden spoon. Pour in the flour gently until the mixture can be rolled by hand, and then put the mixture on a board or countertop that has been a bit dusted with flour to prevent it from sticking. Dust your hands with flour as well and then work the flour into the butter mixture until it starts to fall apart and not stick together.

3. Next, put the mixture on a cookie sheet or heavy steel baking pan, and evenly spread it to cover the whole pan. Pierce multiple times with a fork. Bake for about 30 minutes until it turns golden brown. Set aside to cool. Slice at once and serve.

Crusty Buttermilk Cookie

Ingredients

- 4 large eggs
- 1½ cup sugar
- 2 sticks unsalted butter, dissolved and cooled
- 3 tablespoons flour
- 1 unbaked piecrust, store bought or homemade
- Dash of salt
- 2 teaspoons pure vanilla extract
- 1¼ cup buttermilk

Preparation

1. Preheat the oven to about 325 degrees F. Mix together the sugar, flour, and salt in a medium mixing bowl.

2. Whisk together the butter and eggs in a big mixing bowl until thoroughly mixed. Stir in the buttermilk and vanilla and keep on whisking. Slowly stir in the flour mixture until all the ingredients have been added.

3. Transfer the filling into the piecrust and bake for an hour. The pie should be entirely set and the top a light golden brown color. Let it cool fully before serving. Sprinkle with powdered sugar, if preferred.

Oven Baked Parmesan Chips

Ingredients

• 5 ounces Parmesan

Preparation

Preheat the oven to about 425 degrees F. use parchment paper or foil to line the inside of a baking sheet. Shred the Parmesan into a mixing bowl. Spread 4 tablespoons of the Parmesan on the baking sheet in piles with 3-inch diameters. Continue the process until you have 8 piles of Parmesan. Use your fingers to arrange into small circles. Bake for about 20 to 25 minutes or until it is dissolved but not bubbly. Take out of the oven and allow it to cool.

Chocolate Whittle Pies

Ingredients

- 3 cups milk chocolate chips
- 2 cups unsalted butter, melted
- ¾ cup granulated sugar
- 3 teaspoons vanilla extract
- 3 medium eggs
- 2 cups light brown sugar
- 3 cups all-purpose flour
- 1½ teaspoon baking soda
- 2 teaspoons baking powder
- 1 teaspoon salt

Preparation

1. Preheat the oven to about 350 degrees F. Line parchment paper inside a baking sheet.

2. Mix the butter and sugars together in a small mixing bowl, stir until it turns fluffy with a pale yellow color and light. Stir in the eggs one by one, and then the vanilla until completely mixed.

3. Combine the baking powder, flour, baking soda and salt together in a different mixing bowl. Gently add the dry ingredients into the bowl of wet ingredients. Pour in the chocolate chips. Divide 2 tablespoons of dough for each

cookie and roll into a ball, giving the dough balls 2-inche spaces apart on the baking sheet.

4. Bake dough for about 15 minutes until the edges begin to turn brown. Remove and place on a wire rack and allow it to cool.

Beef And Herbs Pudding

Ingredients

• 1½ cups all-purpose flour

• 4 large eggs

• 4 tablespoons diced fresh mixed herbs such as chives, thyme, and parsley

• 1½ cups milk

• ½ cup reserved beef drippings or dissolved butter

• Freshly ground black pepper and kosher salt

Preparation

1. Preheat the oven to about 475 degrees F.

2. Put an 8 by 12-inch cast iron baking dish in the preheated oven for about 10 minutes. Next, whisk the eggs in a small mixing bowl until it is fluffy and light. Stir in the milk and combine. Pour in the flour, a big pinch of salt, herbs, and some pepper, stir until the batter becomes smooth. Transfer the beef drippings to the hot pan. Next, pour in the batter and bake for roughly 10 minutes. Lower the oven temperature to around 350 degrees F and keep on baking for another 15 to 20 minutes until the pudding becomes brown and puffy. Serve at once.

Bread And Apple Pudding

Ingredients

- 7 eggs
- 7 cups 1/2-inch diced challah bread
- 2 cups milk
- 4 large Granny Smith apples, skinned, cored and chopped
- 1½ tablespoon butter
- 2 cups cream
- 2 teaspoons vanilla extract
- 3 tablespoons honey
- ½ teaspoon ground cinnamon
- ½ teaspoon salt
- Powdered sugar, for dusting
- ½ teaspoon ground nutmeg

Preparation

1. Grease a 2-quart baking dish with butter. Combine the diced bread and apples in a big mixing bowl, and arrange them uniformly in the baking dish.

2. Combine the cream, eggs, milk, vanilla, honey, cinnamon, salt and nutmeg together in a medium-sized bowl. Stir in the liquid mixture on top of the bread and apples. Refrigerate for approximately 2 hours.

3. Preheat the oven to about 375 degrees F.

4. Place the baking dish in a bigger metal roasting pan. Transfer hot water into the roasting pan until it is about 1-inch high in the baking dish. Bake for about 1 to 2 hours until the pudding becomes set and the top turns golden brown. Allow it to cool a bit, sprinkle powdered sugar on it and serve.

Crusty Chocolate Cakes

Ingredients

- 5 large eggs, at room temperature
- 3 cups diced white chocolate
- 2¼ cups store-bought dulce de leche
- ½ cup butter
- 1 cup all-purpose flour
- ½ cup sugar
- Maldon sea salt, for sprinkling

Preparation

1. Dissolve the butter and the white chocolate in a pan over low heat. Stir in the dulce de leche and whisk until well blended. Remove from the heat and leave to stand.

2. Preheat the oven to around 425 degrees F.

3. With a hand or stand mixer, whisk the eggs and sugar until the mixture turns pale and has increased in quantity. Gently stir in the white chocolate mixture and the flour. Stir properly to avoid lumps.

4. Split the batter into 6 ramekins and bake the cake for about 15 minutes until they turn to golden brown and the middles are very tender. Spice with sea salt and serve.

Salty Baked Pecan Pie

Ingredients

- 4 big eggs, lightly whisked
- 2 deep-dish frozen pie crusts
- 1 1/3 cup light corn syrup
- 1½ tablespoon flaky sea salt, for garnish
- 1¼ cup packed dark brown sugar
- 3 cups pecans, shredded
- 7 tablespoons unsalted butter, cut into pieces

Preparation

1. Preheat the oven to about 375 degrees F.

2. Arrange the piecrust on a baking sheet, pierce with a fork and bake for about 15 to 20 minutes.

3. Pour the corn syrup, brown sugar, butter and salt into a medium-sized saucepan. Place on medium heat and stir the mixture as it dissolves. Allow it to boil. Turn off the heat and leave it to cool. Stir in the pecans and the eggs. Place the pie shell on the baking sheet and bake for about an hour. Leave to cool properly before serving.

Buttery Almond Shortbread Cookies

Ingredients

- 2 medium eggs

- 10 ounces natural skin-on almonds

- 5 cups all-purpose flour, sifted

- 2 small (1-ounce) bottle almond extract

- 1½ cups sugar

- 1 pound unsalted butter, at room temperature

Preparation

1. Preheat the oven to about 375 degrees F.

2. Use a food processor to blend the almonds to very smooth crumbs. Pour into a bowl and sprinkle over half of the almond extract. Whisk to mix properly.

3. Whisk together the sugar and butter in a big mixing bowl, using an electric mixer on medium-high speed, until it becomes fluffy, light, and pale yellow. Whisk in the eggs until it is blended together. Stir in the ground almonds, flour, and the rest of the almond extract on low speed. The dough would be very stiff.

4. Mould the dough into shortbread tins, about two-thirds full. Bake for about 10 to 15 minutes in batches if necessary, until it turns a golden brown and sets. Remove the pans and

cool for another 10 minutes, and then gradually empty from the tins.

Creamy Cheese Piecrust

Ingredients

GRAHAM CRACKER CRUST:

- 7 tablespoons unsalted butter, dissolved

- 2 cups graham cracker crumbs

- 2 teaspoons powdered cinnamon

- ½ cup confectioners' sugar

CREAM CHEESE FILLING:

3 medium eggs, at room temperature

15 ounces cream cheese, at room temperature

3 teaspoons vanilla extract

1¼ cup granulated sugar

SOUR CREAM TOPPING:

4 tablespoons granulated sugar

1½ cup sour cream

1½ teaspoon vanilla extract

Preparations

1. To make the graham cracker crust: Preheat the oven to about 375 degrees F.

2. Mix together the graham cracker crumbs with the dissolved butter, cinnamon and confectioners' sugar in a

small mixing bowl. Pour into a 9-inch pie pan and bake for about 10 to 12 minutes. Allow to cool properly before filling.

3. To make the cream cheese filling: Pour the granulated sugar, cream cheese, eggs and vanilla into a medium-sized mixing bowl and whisk with a hand mixer on medium speed until it becomes smooth. Empty the filling into the cooled crust and bake for about 15 to 25 minutes until it sets. Allow to cool for 5 minutes before topping.

4. To make the sour cream topping: mix together the granulated sugar, sour cream and vanilla in a small mixing bowl and stir until smooth. Spread mixture onto the pie and bake for about 10 to 15 minutes. Leave to cool to room temperature and then freeze for about 4 hours. Cut and serve.

Roasted Spiced Carrots

Ingredients

• 4 pounds real baby carrots or regular carrots, sliced into matchsticks

• 4 tablespoons brown sugar

• ½ cup olive oil

• Dash chili powder

• 2 tablespoons cumin

• Kosher salt

Preparation

Preheat the oven to about 400 degrees F.

Combine the olive oil, cumin, brown sugar and chili powder together in a mixing bowl; spice with salt. Flip the carrots in the flavored oil, and then lay those on a foil- or parchment-lined baking sheet. Bake for about 30 to 50 minutes or until it turns brown and softens.

Baked Vanilla Meringues

Ingredients

- 2 teaspoon vanilla, orange flower water, or maple extract
- 5 egg whites
- 1 cup sugar
- ¼ teaspoon cream of tartar
- 1¼ tablespoon cornstarch
- ¾ cup icing sugar
- Dash salt

Preparation

1. Preheat the oven to 225 degrees F.

2. Beat the egg whites and salt in a clean mixing bowl until soft peaks appear, stir in the vanilla, and keep on whisking to stiff peaks. Pour the cream of tartar into the regular sugar and beat it into the egg whites mixture very gently, a spoonful at a time, until the meringue becomes stiff and the sugar melts. Sift together the cornstarch and icing sugar. Sift over the meringue and gradually pour in until fully blended.

3. Spoon the meringues onto a baking sheet lined with parchment. Bake for an hour to two or until it turns cream-colored and crisp on top when tapped. Take it out of the oven and leave it to cool on the trays. Store in a sealed container till ready to serve.

Baked Cheese Pasta

Ingredients

- 2 big eggs
- 1 to 2 sticks unsalted butter
- 2½ cups milk
- 3 cups sharp Cheddar, shredded
- One, 12-ounce box dry elbow macaroni
- Ground black pepper
- Paprika, for garnishing
- Salt

Preparation

1. Preheat the oven to about 375 degrees F. Gently grease a 9- by 13-inch baking dish.

2. Boil the elbow macaroni in a big pot of salted water until it is 4 minutes from being fully done. Drain the water and stir in the cheese and butter, and spice with pepper and salt. Flip until the butter is dissolved and all are well mixed. Transfer into the selected baking dish.

3. Beat the egg and milk together in a big mixing bowl. Drain the mixture into the pot of pasta and stir together. Garnish with the paprika.

4. Uncover and bake for half an hour until the top turns brown. Serve at once.

Creamy Cornbread

Ingredients

- 3 eggs
- 3 cups yellow cornmeal
- 1¼ cup buttermilk
- 1½ tablespoon sugar
- 3 tablespoons canola oil
- 1 teaspoon baking soda
- 3 teaspoons baking powder
- 1¼ cup creamed corn
- 1½ teaspoon kosher salt

Preparation

1. Preheat the oven to about 425 degrees F.

2. Put a 10-inch cast iron skillet inside the oven.

3. Mix together the sugar, cornmeal, baking powder, salt, and baking soda in a mixing bowl. Stir together to mix properly.

4. In a large bowl, mix together the eggs, buttermilk, and creamed corn in a mixing bowl and stir together to mix thoroughly. Stir the dry ingredients into the bowl of buttermilk mixture and mix properly. If the batter is too thick, stir in more buttermilk.

5. Twirl the canola oil in the hot cast iron skillet to spread evenly. Transfer the batter into the skillet and bake for about 20 minutes until the cornbread turns golden brown and rises back upon when pushed down slightly.

Wine And Tomato Sauce

Ingredients

- 25 Roma tomatoes, halved and seeded
- 1¼ cup white wine
- ½ cup olive oil
- 1½ teaspoon pepper
- 2 teaspoons garlic, chopped
- 1¼ cup thinly sliced onion
- 2 tablespoons thyme leaves, thinly diced
- 2 tablespoons oregano leaves, thinly sliced
- 1 teaspoon kosher salt

Preparation

Preheat the oven to about 325 degrees F.

Arrange the tomato halves side up in 2 (13 by 9-inch) pans. Pour in the oil, salt, onion, herbs, garlic and pepper. Bake the tomatoes for about 2 hours. Inspect the tomatoes after 60 minutes and lower the heat if they appear to be cooking too fast. Then increase the oven heat to 400 degrees and bake for another half hour. Take out the trays from the oven and process the tomatoes through a food mill on medium dye setting over a medium-sized saucepan. Dispose of the skins. Stir in the white wine, allow it to boil, lower the heat to a simmer and cook for another 5 minutes.

Bread With Sweet Corn Pudding

Ingredients

- 3 cups diced French bread
- 1 large onion, thinly chopped
- 1 (15-ounce) can creamed style sweet corn
- 1 ounce unsalted butter
- 3 eggs
- 1 teaspoon rosemary
- 1 teaspoon thyme
- 1¼ cup heavy cream
- ¾ cup yellow cornmeal, whole grain, stone ground
- 1¼ teaspoon baking powder
- 1¼ teaspoon kosher salt
- 1 cup Parmesan, shredded
- Ground black pepper

Preparation

1. Heat the oven to about 350 degrees F.

2. Sweat the onions with the herbs and butter in an oven-safe skillet until becomes lucent.

3. Mix together the cream, cornmeal, salt, corn, baking powder, eggs, Parmesan, and pepper in a big mixing bowl. Top with diced bread and toss to mix. Transfer the batter

into the skillet, directly on the onion mixture. Bake for close to an hour, or until it sets firmly. Allow it to cool a bit before serving.

Buttery Cocoa Cookies

Ingredients

- Flour, for dusting buttered pan
- 10 ounces dissolved butter
- 5 big eggs
- Soft butter, for greasing the pan
- 1¼ cup brown sugar, sifted
- 1¼ cup sugar, sifted
- 1 cup flour, sifted
- 3 teaspoons vanilla extract
- 1½ cups cocoa, sifted
- 1 teaspoon kosher salt

Preparation

1. Preheat the oven to about 300 degrees F. Rub butter and flour into an 8-inch square pan.

2. Whisk the eggs at medium speed until they become light yellow and fluffy using a mixer fitted with a whisk attachment. Stir in both sugars. Pour in the rest of the ingredients, and stir to mix properly.

3. Transfer the batter into a greased and floured 8-inch square pan and bake for roughly 40 minutes. Use a toothpick dipped into the middle of the pan to know if it is done when the toothpick comes out clean. Once done,

transfer to a rack to cool. Don't cut into it until it's completely cool.

Salty Parmesan Brussels Sprouts

Ingredients

• 2 pounds Brussels sprouts, spruced, halved through the stem end

• 3 tablespoons unsalted butter, cut into bits

• 4 tablespoons extra-virgin olive oil

• ¾ cup panko breadcrumbs

• ¾ teaspoon coarse salt

• 3 cloves garlic, finely diced

• ¾ cup ground Parmesan cheese

Preparation

1. Preheat the oven to about 425 degrees F.

2. Boil the Brussels sprouts in a big pot of cooking salted water for about 5 minutes until it is tender but not collapsing. Drain from the water properly.

3. Pour the oil and garlic into a 9- by 13-inch baking pan and sauté for about 3 to 6 minutes until fragrant. Stir in the Brussels sprouts and salt and stir to coat. Mix together the breadcrumbs and the Parmesan in a small mixing bowl and garnish the mixture over the Brussels sprouts. Do it with the butter.

4. Bake for about 15 minutes until the crumbs turn golden brown and the Brussels sprouts become tender and very hot.

Salty Parmesan Biscuits

Ingredients

BISCUITS:

- 3 cups flour
- 1 teaspoon salt
- 1 cup butter
- 2 eggs
- 1¼ teaspoon sugar

TOPPINGS:

Grated coriander seed with 5 spice

Grated dill seed

Paprika and cayenne pepper

Grated fennel seed

Sesame seeds

Poppy seeds

Grated cumin seed and cayenne pepper

Fleur de sel, for sprinkling

Parmesan and herbes de Provence

Mixed peppercorns

Preparation

1. Heat the oven to about 425 degrees F.

2. In a mixing bowl, combine the sugar, butter, salt, eggs and 3 tablespoons of cold water together and mix properly. Stir in the flour and combine promptly until it sets. Do not overwork. Roll the dough into 1/16 of an inch thick. Slice into squares. Garnish with some fleur de sel and any topping you prefer. Place on a baking sheet and bake until it is crisp, puffed, and golden.

Spicy Honeyed Chicken Wings

Ingredients

- 4 pounds chicken wings, chopped, wing tips disposed
- Vegetable oil, for greasing
- 1 teaspoon hot sauce, like Tabasco
- 1 teaspoon freshly ground black pepper
- 2 tablespoon soy sauce
- 4 tablespoons honey
- ¾ teaspoon cumin
- 2 teaspoons curry powder
- Sweet chili sauce, for dipping
- 2 teaspoon kosher salt

Preparation

1. Preheat the oven to about 425 degrees F. Evenly rub oil in 2 baking pans. Flip the wings in the salt and pepper mixture, and then split equally between the pans, allowing enough space between the chicken parts. Bake for about an hour, flipping the wings occasionally and changing the position of the pans occasionally until it turns crisp and a golden brown.

2. Next, combine the soy sauce, honey, cumin, curry powder, and hot sauce in a big mixing bowl. Flip the chicken wings to coat, and then place in one of the pans and keep on baking

until it is glazed and burnt in places. Serve with a little bowl of sweet chili sauce, for dipping.

If you enjoyed reading this book please endeavor to leave a positive review at the customer review section below.

ABOUT THE AUTHOR

After a long successful career tutoring some of the best culinary schools in the states, Virginia Anne Caldwell has retired to her home in the country side where she continues to prepare and teach some of the best recipes and cooking lessons to family members and friends.
With extensive knowledge accumulated over the years on the art of cooking, Virginia continues to share her secrets on various blogs and cookbooks.

For more of my awesome cookbooks and recipes please visit my author central page:

amazon.com/author/virginiacaldwell

BAKING DEMYSTIFIED

50 Easy And Delicious Grain-Free And Gluten-Free Baking Recipes: (Weight watchers Cooking 2)

Making lifestyle changes that foster better health in order to be more physically active, improve stress management and cultivate a healthy diet doesn't include giving up on those superfoods that you enjoy eating.

FACT: One of the best ways to lower fat consumption is to switch from deep-fried foods to baked foods. Baking requires little or no oil and as such is the ideal choice for weight management.

BAKING DEMYSTIFIED: contains about 50 Easy and Delicious Grain-Free and Gluten-Free Baking Recipes with step-by-step instructions for the preparation of breads, biscuits, muffins and lots of other savory dishes for you and your family including:

- Baked Scottish Bread
- Baked Salmon with Truffles in Puff Pastry
- Fat-free Chocolate Cookies
- Baked Cheesy Tortellini Sauce
- Sweet Bacon Soufflé
- Oven Baked Crusty Pumpkin Cheesecake
- Baked Barbeque Bean Sauce

Most of these meals can be prepared within 10 to 30 minutes making them the perfect choice for breakfast, lunch or dinner as well as on special occasions like thanksgiving.